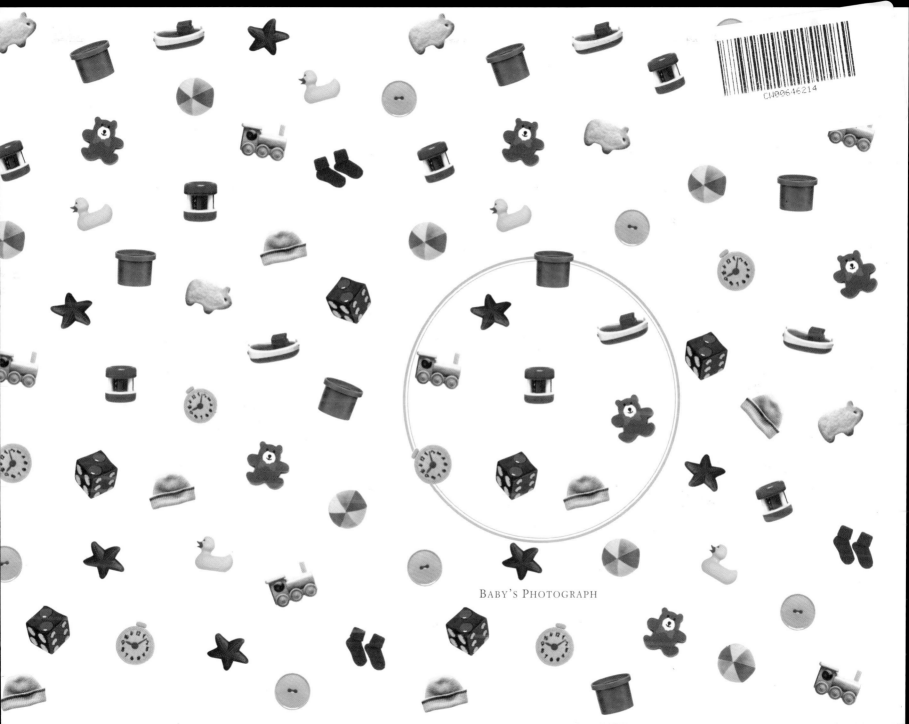

BABY'S PHOTOGRAPH

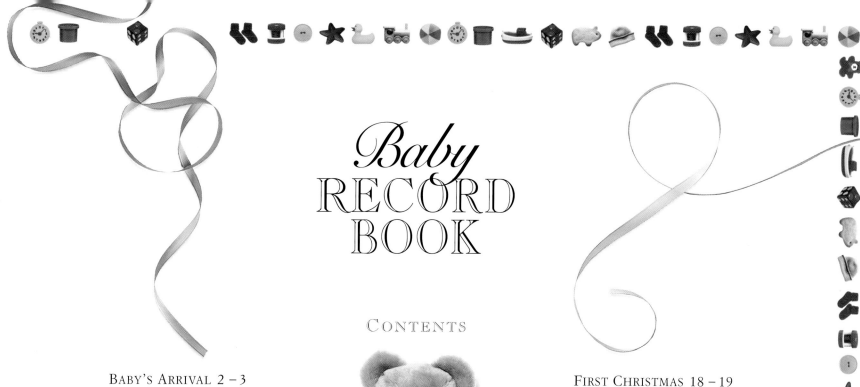

Baby
RECORD
BOOK

CONTENTS

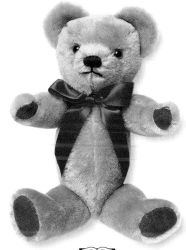

DORLING KINDERSLEY
London • New York • Stuttgart

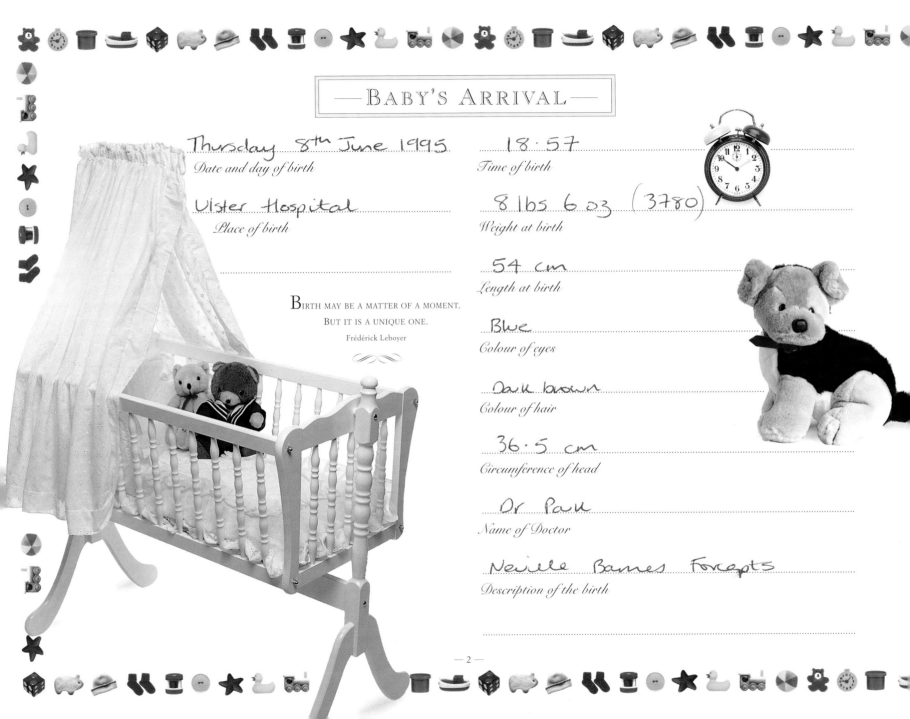

BABY'S ARRIVAL

Thursday 8th June 1995
Date and day of birth

Ulster Hospital
Place of birth

Birth may be a matter of a moment.
But it is a unique one.
Frédérick Leboyer

18·57
Time of birth

8 lbs 6 oz (3780)
Weight at birth

54 cm
Length at birth

Blue
Colour of eyes

Dark brown
Colour of hair

36·5 cm
Circumference of head

Dr Paul
Name of Doctor

Neville Barnes Forceps
Description of the birth

— 2 —

Beautiful !

Baby's appearance

Birth cards received

Monday's child is fair of face,
Tuesday's child is full of grace,
Wednesday's child is full of woe,
Thursday's child has far to go,
Friday's child is loving and giving,
Saturday's child works hard for a living,
And the child that is born on the Sabbath day
Is bonny and blithe, and good and gay.

Horoscope

Zodiac sign

Chinese horoscope

Birthstone

Flower

BIRTH ANNOUNCEMENT

FIRST DAYS

First visitors

Nanna, Pappa, Michael, Carolyn and
Reuben

Anty Margaret, Granny and Uncle Allan,
Cindy, Clifford and Debbie,
Alastair & Joanne, Rosemany
and Philip.

Their comments

" Very distinguished."
" Gorgeous baby."
" He's like Andrew."

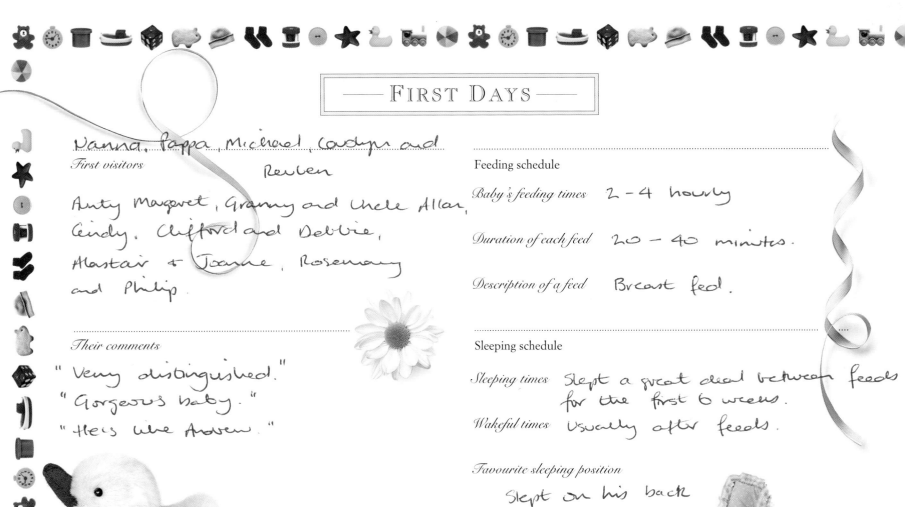

A BABE IS FED WITH MILK AND PRAISE.

Charles and Mary Lamb

Feeding schedule

Baby's feeding times   2 - 4 hourly

Duration of each feed   20 - 40 minutes.

Description of a feed   Breast fed.

Sleeping schedule

Sleeping times   Slept a great deal between feeds
for the first 6 weeks.

Wakeful times   Usually after feeds.

Favourite sleeping position
Slept on his back

Mother's feelings
Delighted. Overwhelmed

Father's feelings

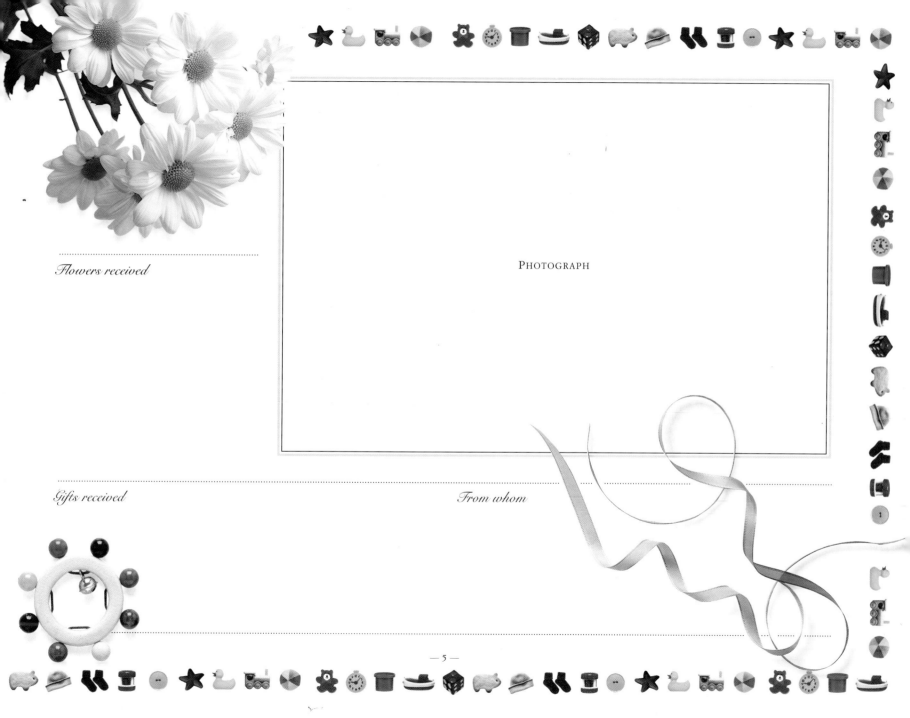

Flowers received

....

PHOTOGRAPH

Gifts received

From whom

NAME CEREMONY

INVITATION

Gifts received

Your baby's behaviour

Reason for choosing name

Description of ceremony

Your baby's outfit

G IVING A NAME IS INDEED A POETIC ART.

Thomas Carlyle

Guests attending

FAMILY TREE

Maternal

Paternal

Great Grandmother

....

....

Great Grandfather

Great Grandmother

....

....

Great Grandfather

Great Grandmother

....

....

Great Grandfather

Great Grandmother

....

....

Great Grandfather

Grandmother

....

....

Grandfather

Grandmother

....

....

Grandfather

Mother

Elizabeth

Father

Sisters

Baby

Daniel

Brothers

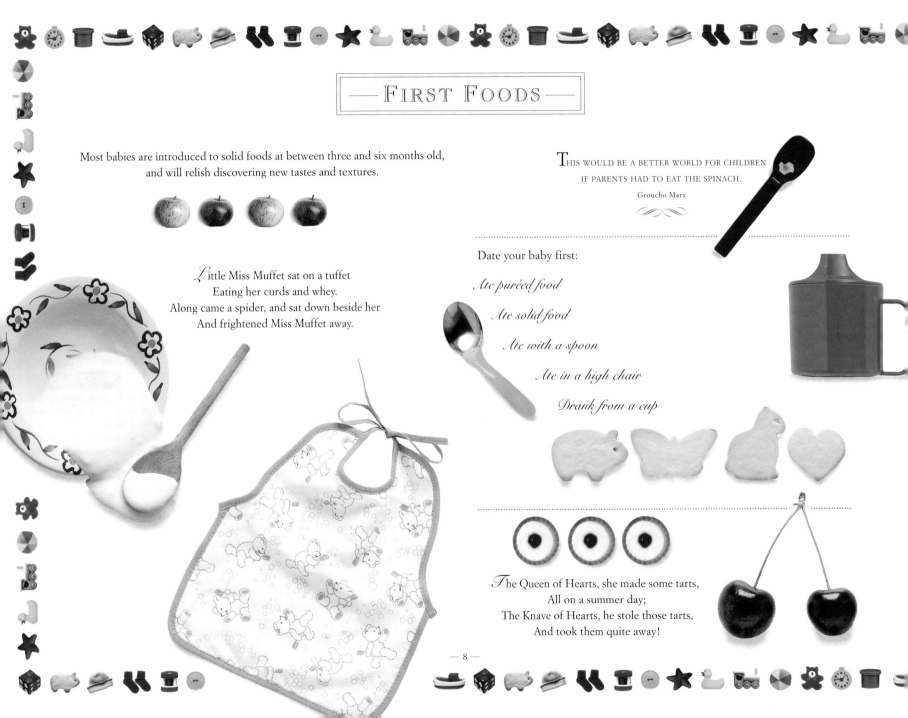

FIRST FOODS

Most babies are introduced to solid foods at between three and six months old, and will relish discovering new tastes and textures.

Little Miss Muffet sat on a tuffet
Eating her curds and whey.
Along came a spider, and sat down beside her
And frightened Miss Muffet away.

THIS WOULD BE A BETTER WORLD FOR CHILDREN IF PARENTS HAD TO EAT THE SPINACH.

Groucho Marx

Date your baby first:

Ate puréed food

Ate solid food

Ate with a spoon

Ate in a high chair

Drank from a cup

The Queen of Hearts, she made some tarts,
All on a summer day;
The Knave of Hearts, he stole those tarts,
And took them quite away!

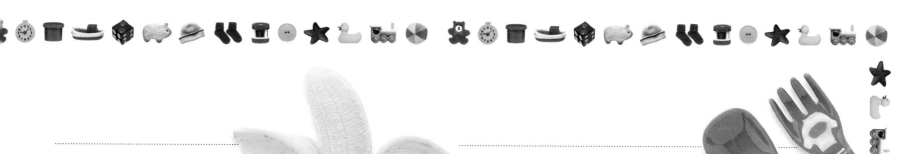

Favourite food

Description of a meal

Date of final feed from breast or bottle

TEETHING

ADAM AND EVE HAD MANY ADVANTAGES, BUT THE PRINCIPAL ONE WAS THAT THEY ESCAPED TEETHING.

Mark Twain

A baby cuts 20 primary or milk teeth, which begin to be replaced with permanent teeth when the child is about six years old. The appearance of the first tooth is a milestone in a baby's life, although it can cause a great deal of discomfort. Some babies find chewing on a teething ring soothes the gums and helps lessen the pain.

Date of first tooth 6/2/96

Date of second tooth 6/2/96

Date of third tooth

Date of fourth tooth

Date of fifth tooth

Teething symptoms

Notes

Top teeth

Teething order

Bottom teeth

PEOPLE WHO SAY THEY SLEEP LIKE A BABY USUALLY DON'T HAVE ONE.

Leo J. Burke

Bedtime

Favourite sleeping position

Wakes at

Bedtime comforters

First sleeps through night

First sleeps in cot

*B*ye, baby bunting,
Daddy's gone a-hunting
Gone to get a rabbit skin
To wrap his baby bunting in.

*S*leep baby, sleep,
Thy father guards the sheep,
Thy mother shakes the dreamland tree,
And from it fall sweet dreams for thee,
Sleep, baby, sleep.

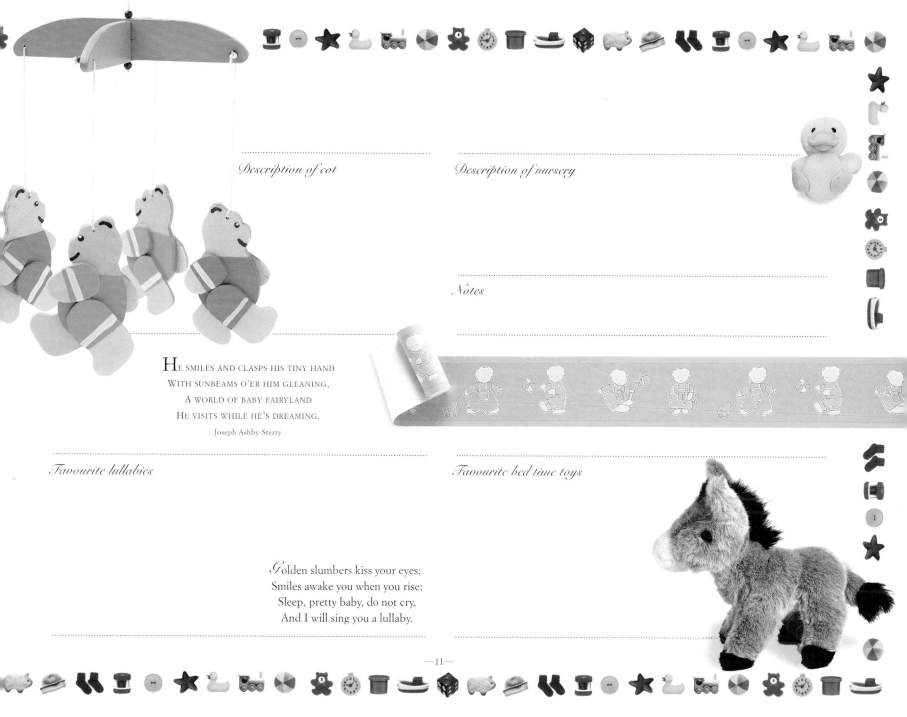

Description of cot

Description of nursery

Notes

He smiles and clasps his tiny hand
With sunbeams o'er him gleaning,
A world of baby fairyland
He visits while he's dreaming.

Joseph Ashby-Sterry

Favourite lullabies

Favourite bed time toys

Golden slumbers kiss your eyes;
Smiles awake you when you rise;
Sleep, pretty baby, do not cry,
And I will sing you a lullaby.

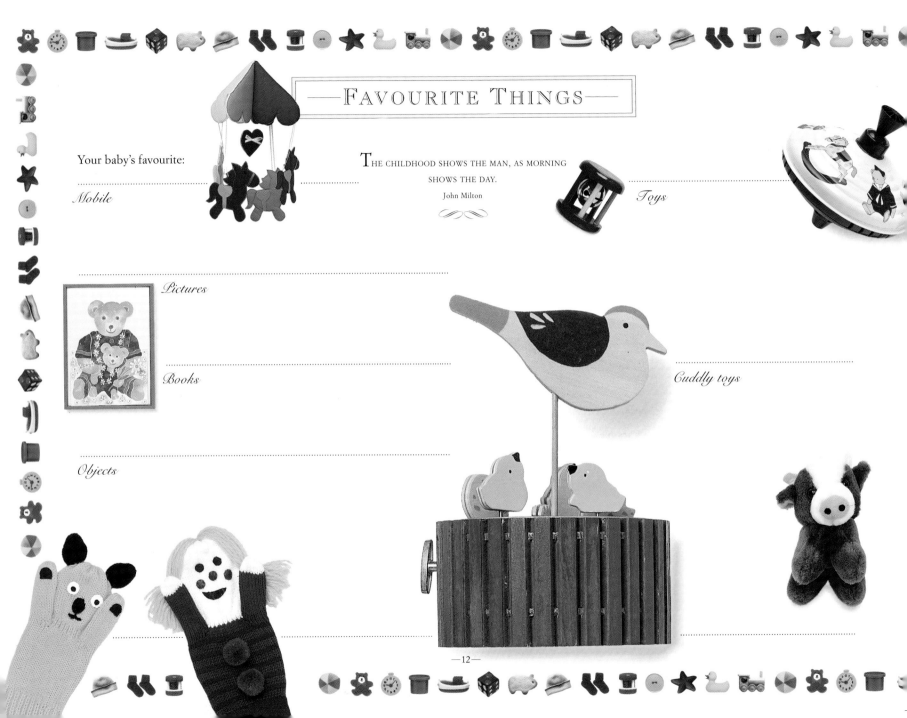

FAVOURITE THINGS

Your baby's favourite:

Mobile

THE CHILDHOOD SHOWS THE MAN, AS MORNING
SHOWS THE DAY.

John Milton

Toys

Pictures

Books

Cuddly toys

Objects

—12—

Games

Activities

Sounds

Words

People

Animals

Stories

Songs and Nursery Rhymes

*H*ey diddle diddle
The cat and the fiddle,
The cow jumped over the moon;
The little dog laughed
To see such sport,
And the dish ran away with the spoon.

— Bathtime and Water Play —

First enjoys bath

....

First time in a big bath

....

Response to being bathed

....

Response to hair being washed

....

I'M VERY FOND OF WATER;
IT EVER MUST DELIGHT
EACH MOTHER'S SON AND DAUGHTER,
WHEN QUALIFIED ARIGHT.

Charles Neaves

Favourite bath toys

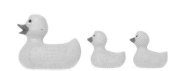

Bath time activities

....

Row, row, row your boat
Gently down the stream
Merrily, merrily, merrily, merrily,
Life is but a dream.

One, two, three, four, five,
Once I caught a fish alive,
Six, seven, eight, nine, ten,
Then I let him go again.
Why did you let him go?
Because he bit my finger so.
Which finger did he bite?
This little finger on the right.

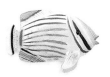
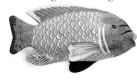

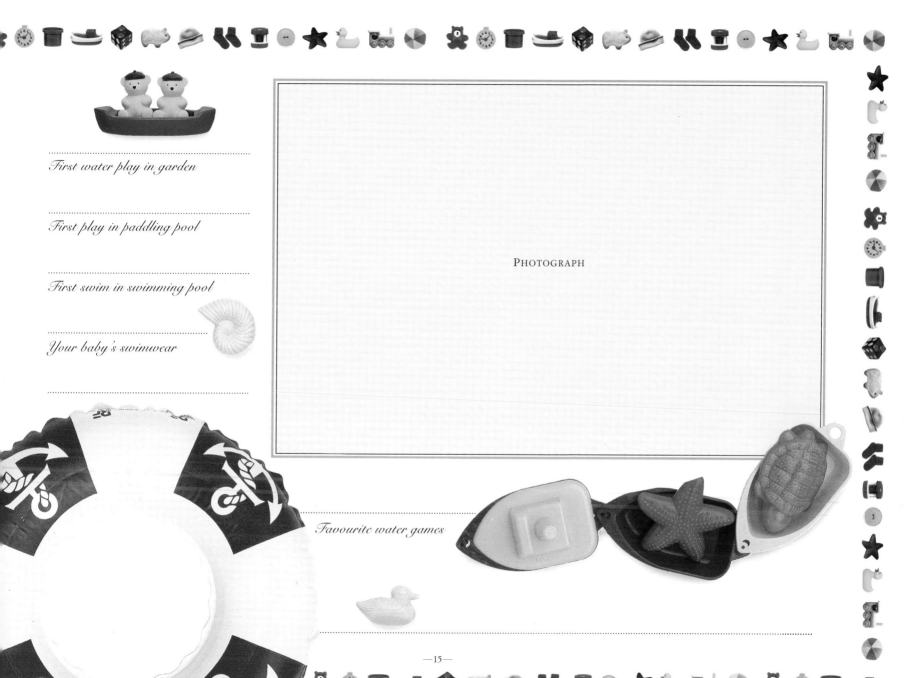

First water play in garden

....

First play in paddling pool

....

First swim in swimming pool

....

Your baby's swimwear

....

PHOTOGRAPH

Favourite water games

FIRST OUTINGS

Details of first journeys made by:

Car

Train

> THERE ARE TWO CLASSES OF TRAVEL –
> FIRST CLASS, AND WITH CHILDREN.
>
> Robert Benchley

Bus

Aeroplane

Boat

Outings to:

Grandparents

Relatives

Special friends

> Ride a cock horse to Banbury Cross,
> To see a fine lady upon a white horse;
> With rings on her fingers, and bells on her toes,
> She shall have music wherever she goes.

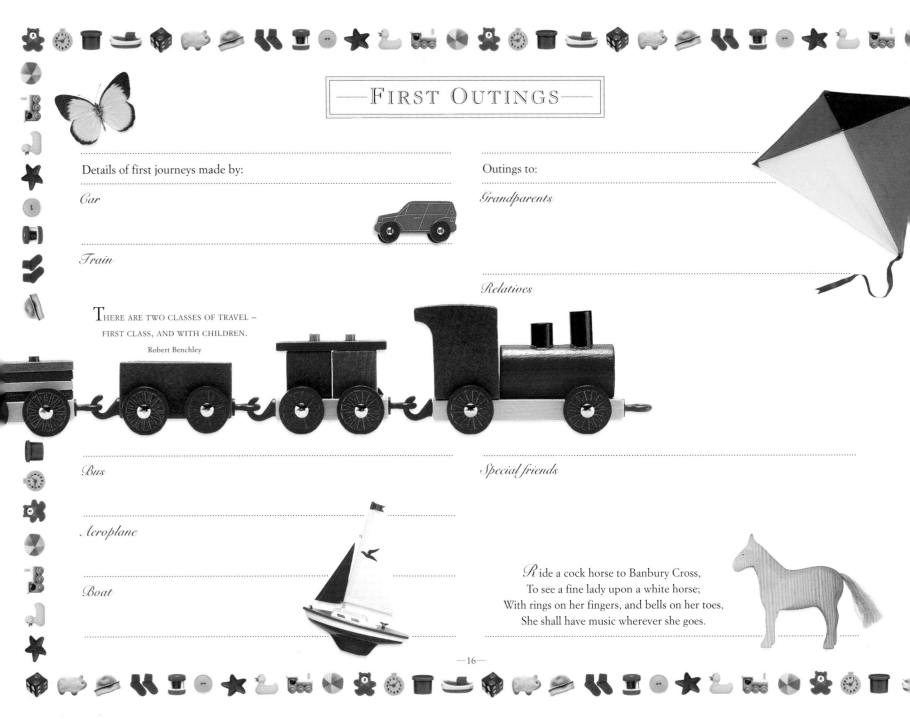

Outings to:

Parks and playgrounds

Beaches

The countryside

Shops

To market, to market,
To buy a fat pig,
Home again, home again,
Jiggetty jig.

Notes

PHOTOGRAPH

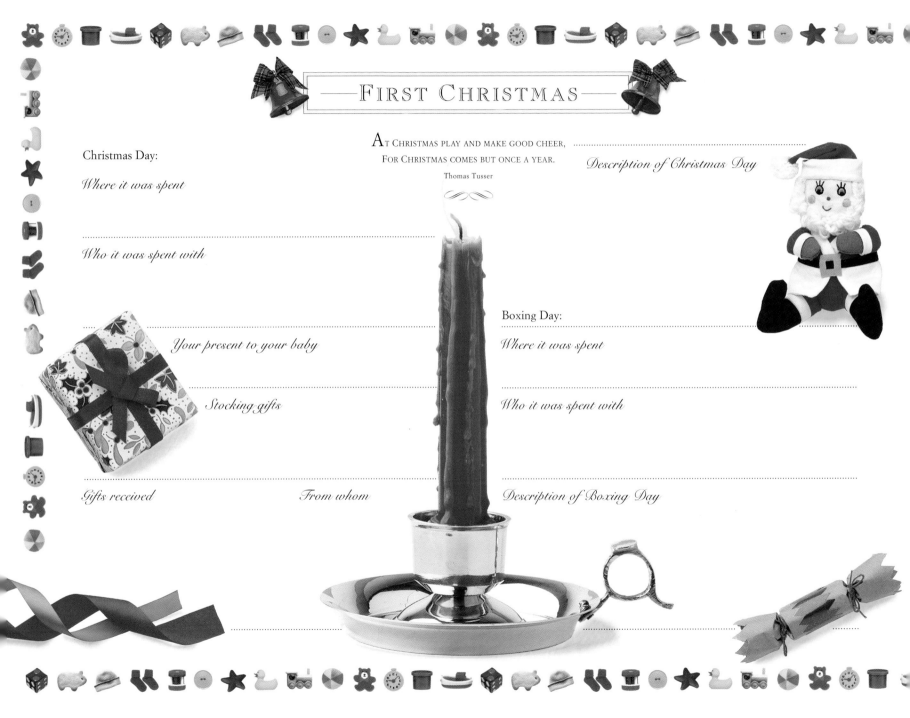

FIRST CHRISTMAS

Christmas Day:

Where it was spent

Who it was spent with

AT CHRISTMAS PLAY AND MAKE GOOD CHEER,
FOR CHRISTMAS COMES BUT ONCE A YEAR.

Thomas Tusser

Description of Christmas Day

Your present to your baby

Stocking gifts

Boxing Day:

Where it was spent

Who it was spent with

Gifts received

From whom

Description of Boxing Day

Favourite Christmas presents

Family Christmas activities

Favourite Christmas games

Description of the Christmas tree

Christmas weather

PHOTOGRAPH

Notes

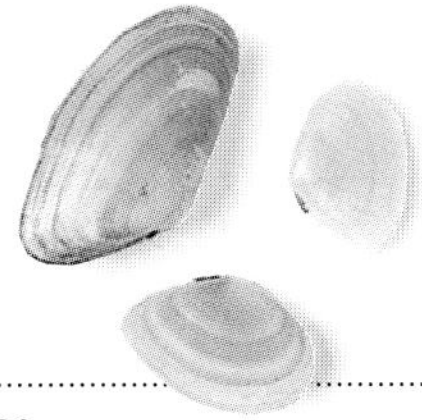

FIRST HOLIDAY

Date

Place

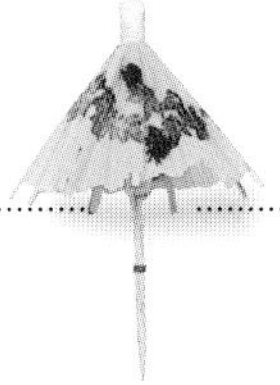

Who was there

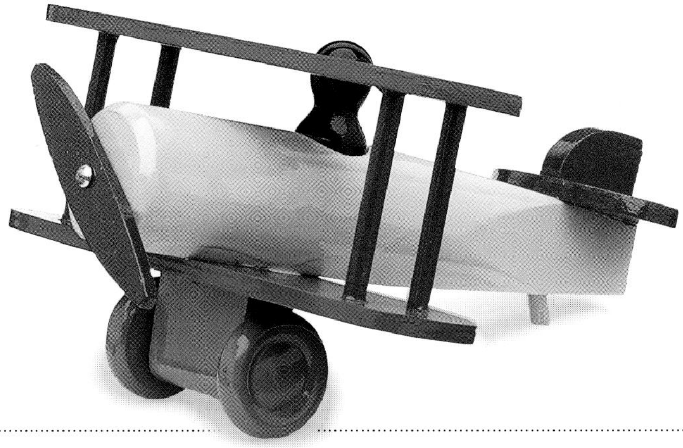

Travel details

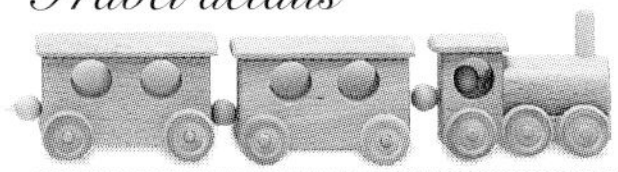

Accommodation

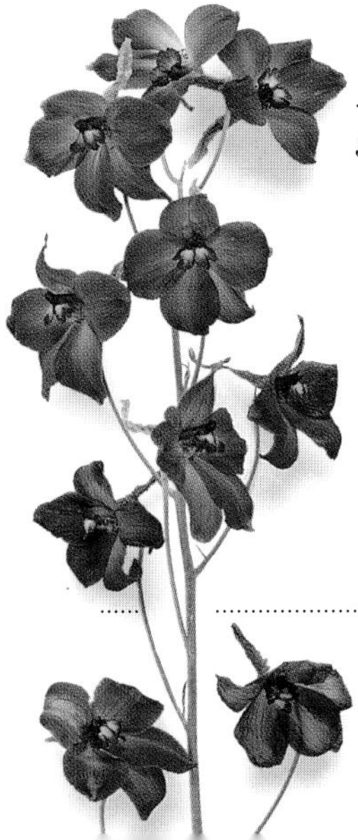

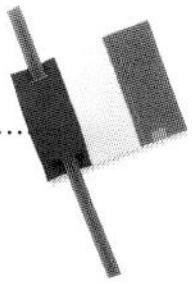

Favourite activities

Favourite outings

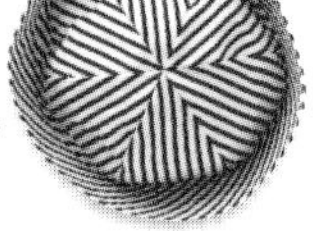

Baby's behaviour

Baby's new friends

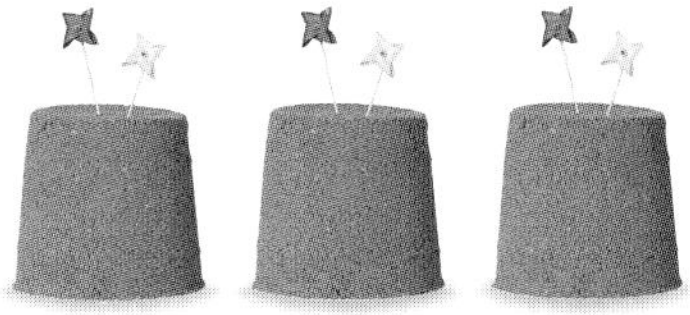

PHOTOGRAPH

Favourite memories of the holiday

Iᴛ ɪs ᴀ ʜᴀᴘᴘʏ ᴛᴀʟᴇɴᴛ ᴛᴏ ᴋɴᴏᴡ ʜᴏᴡ ᴛᴏ ᴘʟᴀʏ.

Ralph Waldo Emerson

FIRST BIRTHDAY

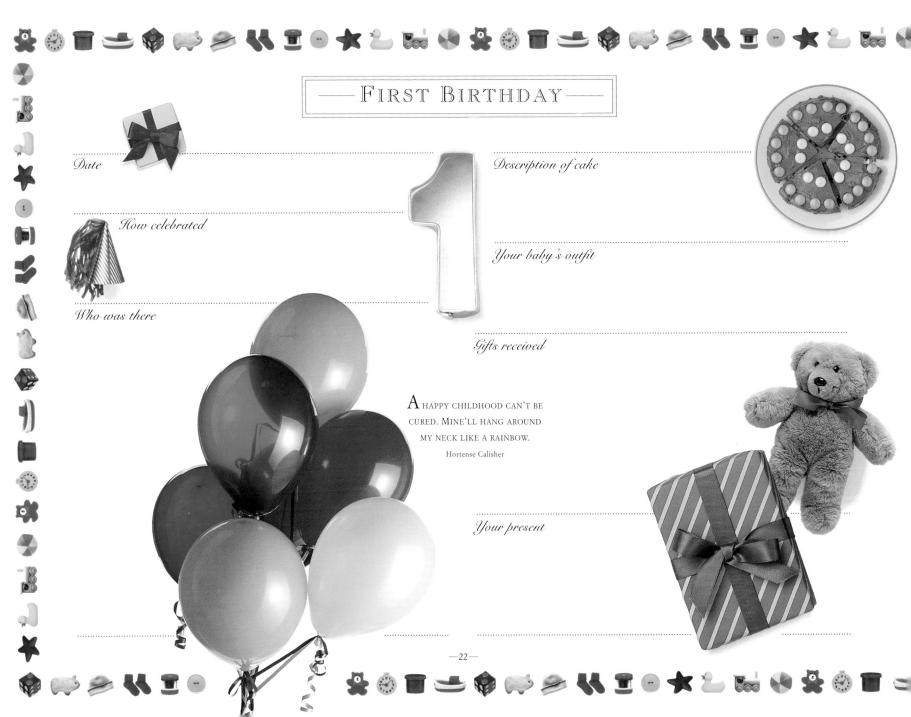

Date

How celebrated

Who was there

Description of cake

Your baby's outfit

Gifts received

A HAPPY CHILDHOOD CAN'T BE
CURED. MINE'LL HANG AROUND
MY NECK LIKE A RAINBOW.
Hortense Calisher

Your present

Your baby's behaviour

*H*appy birthday to you
Happy birthday to you
Happy birthday dear baby
Happy birthday to you.

PHOTOGRAPH

Notes

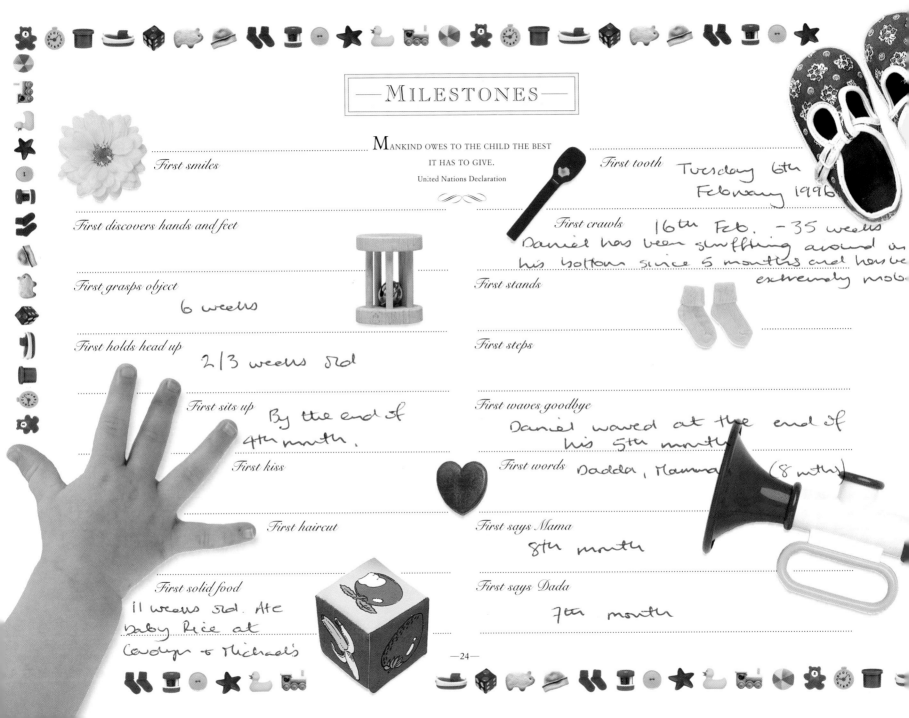

─ MILESTONES ─

MANKIND OWES TO THE CHILD THE BEST
IT HAS TO GIVE.

United Nations Declaration

First smiles

First discovers hands and feet

First grasps object

6 weeks

First holds head up

2/3 weeks old

First sits up

By the end of 4th month.

First kiss

First haircut

First solid food

11 weeks old. Ate baby Rice at Carolyn & Michael's

First tooth

Tuesday 6th February 1996

First crawls

16th Feb. - 35 weeks Daniel has been shuffling around on his bottom since 5 months and has been extremely mobile

First stands

First steps

First waves goodbye

Daniel waved at the end of his 5th month

First words Dadda, Mamma (8 mths)

First says Mama

8th month

First says Dada

7th month

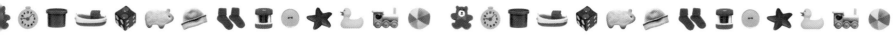

We FIND DELIGHT IN THE BEAUTY AND
HAPPINESS OF CHILDREN THAT MAKES THE
HEART TOO BIG FOR THE BODY.

Ralph Waldo Emerson

....

First recognizes:

Mother

Father

Grandparents

Special friends

Animals

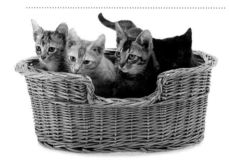

First friends

PHOTOGRAPH

....

Notes

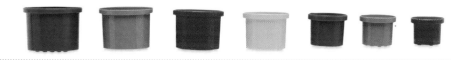

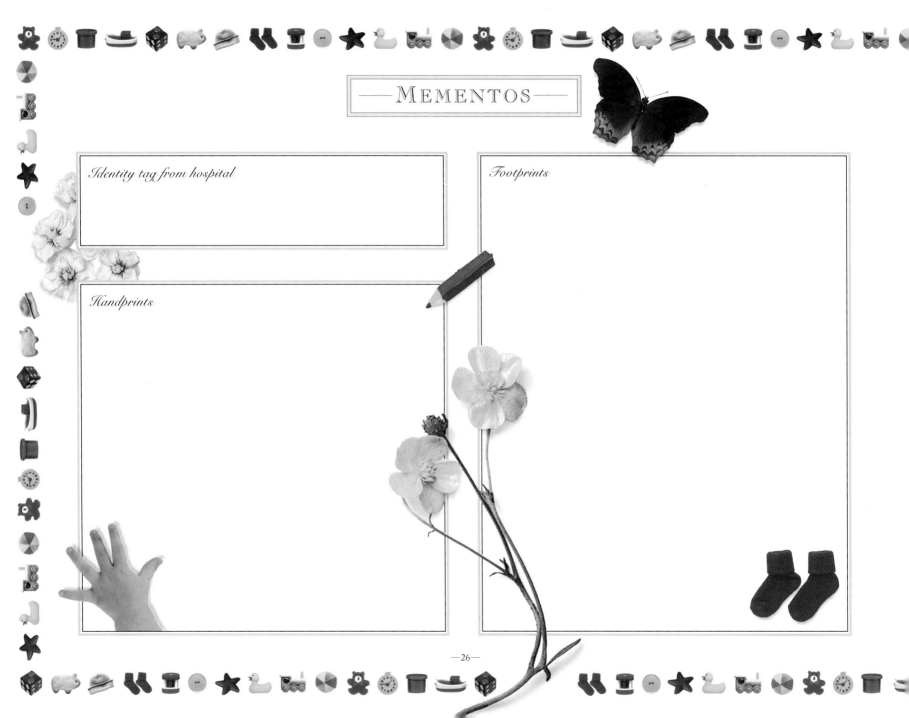

MEMENTOS

Identity tag from hospital

Footprints

Handprints

—26—

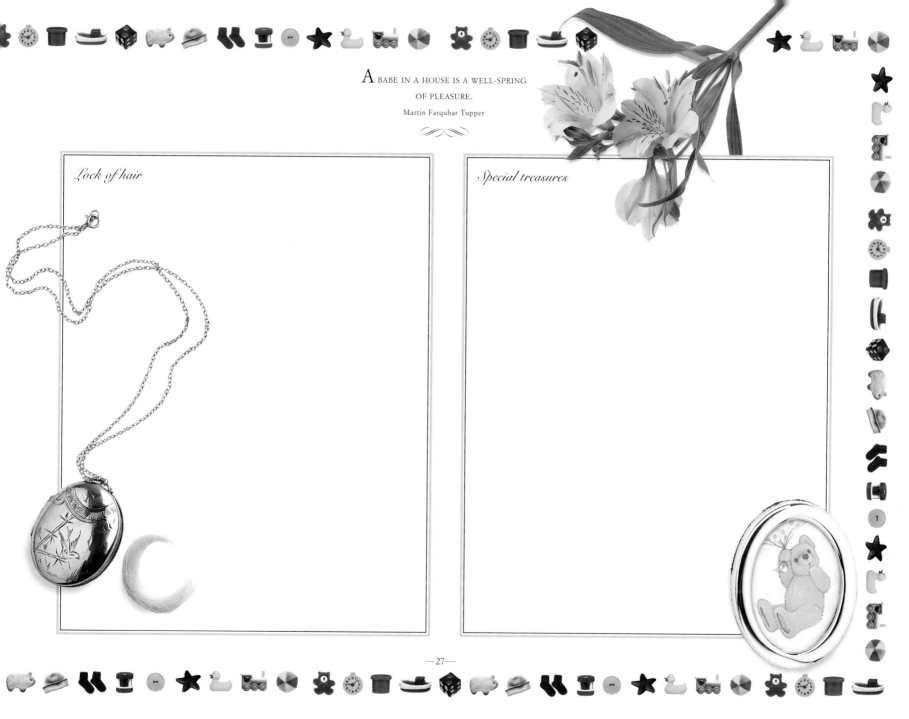

A BABE IN A HOUSE IS A WELL-SPRING
OF PLEASURE.

Martin Farquhar Tupper

Lock of hair

Special treasures

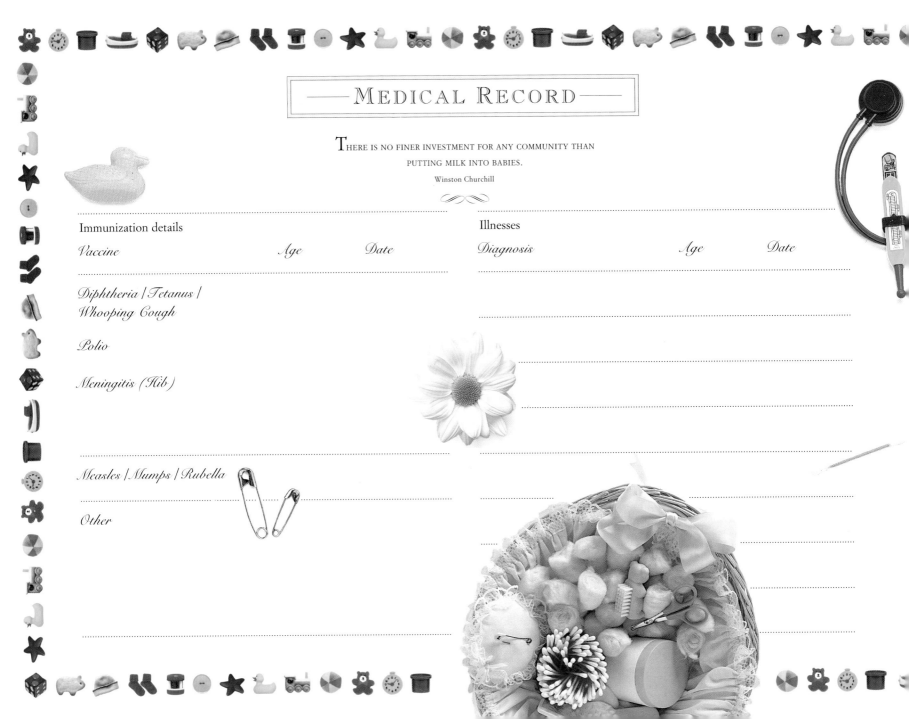

Medical Record

There is no finer investment for any community than
putting milk into babies.

Winston Churchill

Immunization details

Vaccine	Age	Date
Diphtheria / Tetanus / *Whooping Cough*		
Polio		
Meningitis (Hib)		
Measles / Mumps / Rubella		
Other		

Illnesses

Diagnosis	Age	Date

Visits to doctor

Reason	Age	Date

Allergies

Blood group

Eyesight test

Hearing test

AGE AND WEIGHT CHART

Weight
Age in months

| lbs | kgs | 0 | 1 | 2 | 3 | 4 | 5 | 6 | 7 | 8 | 9 | 10 | 11 | 12 |

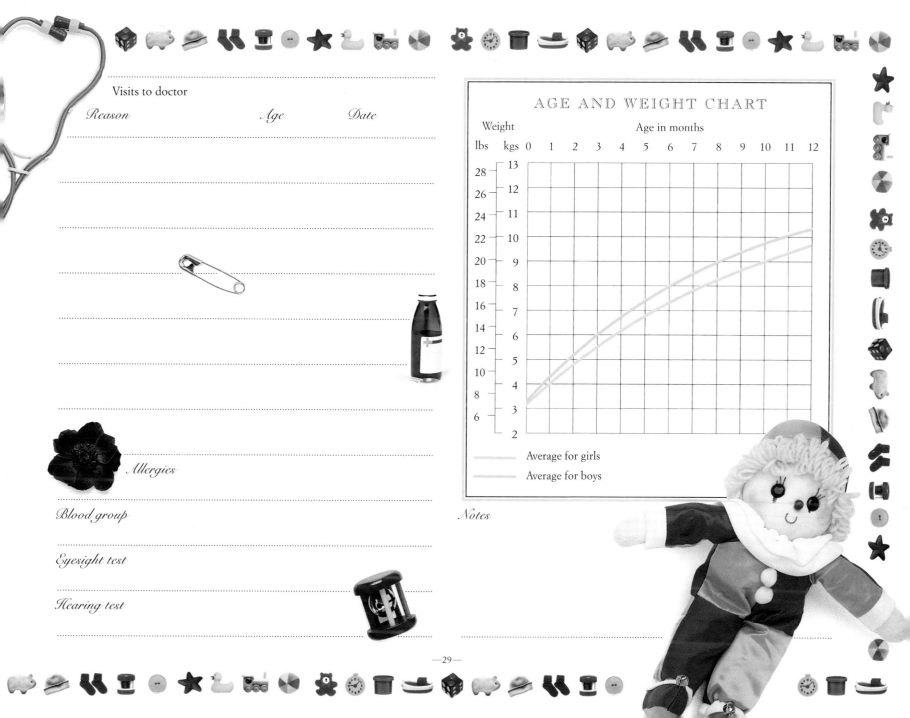

———— Average for girls
———— Average for boys

Notes

SPECIAL MEMORIES

Of all the wonderful things to have happened during your baby's first year of
life, some will stand out as particularly memorable and worth recording.

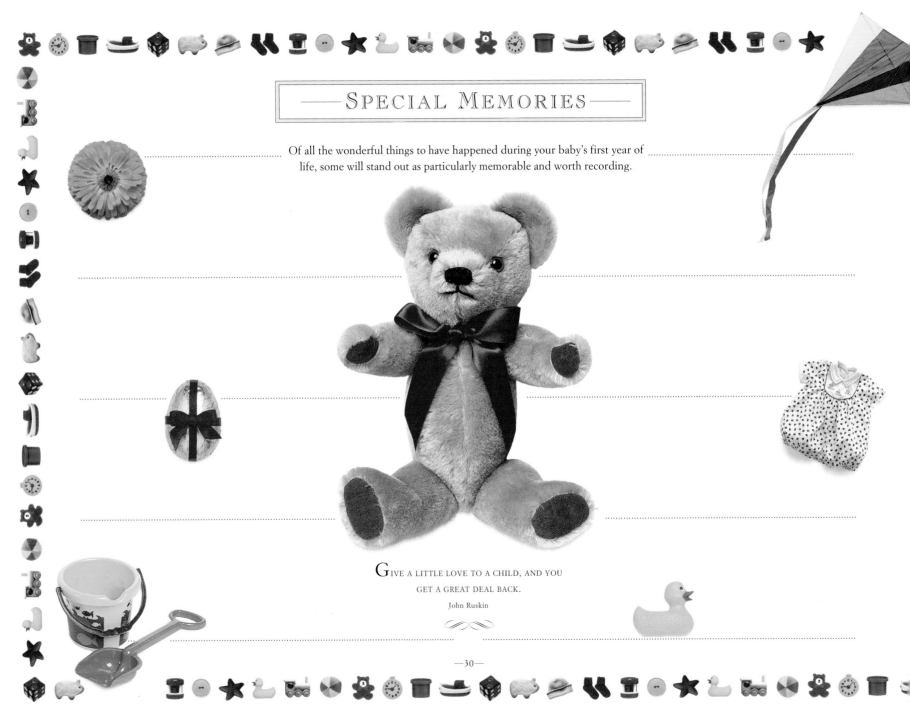

GIVE A LITTLE LOVE TO A CHILD, AND YOU

GET A GREAT DEAL BACK.

John Ruskin

HOPES FOR THE FUTURE

....

Plans for the future

....

Possible schools

....

Prediction of future occupation

....

Your baby's character

PERHAPS A CHILD WHO IS FUSSED OVER GETS A FEELING
OF DESTINY, HE THINKS HE IS IN THE WORLD FOR SOMETHING
IMPORTANT AND IT GIVES HIM DRIVE AND CONFIDENCE.

Benjamin Spock

PHOTOGRAPH

FROM 8/6   TO 8/7

DAY 1	DAY 2	DAY 3	DAY 4		DAY 5	
Date 8/6/95						HOMECOMING
DAY 7	DAY 8	DAY 9	DAY 10	DAY 11	DAY 12	DAY 13
DAY 14	DAY 15	DAY 16	DAY 17	DAY 18	DAY 19	DAY 20
	DAY 21	DAY 22	DAY 23	DAY 24	DAY 25	DAY 26
	DAY 27	DAY 28	DAY 29	DAY 30	DAY 31	

Don't forget – start using the stickers to record your baby's development

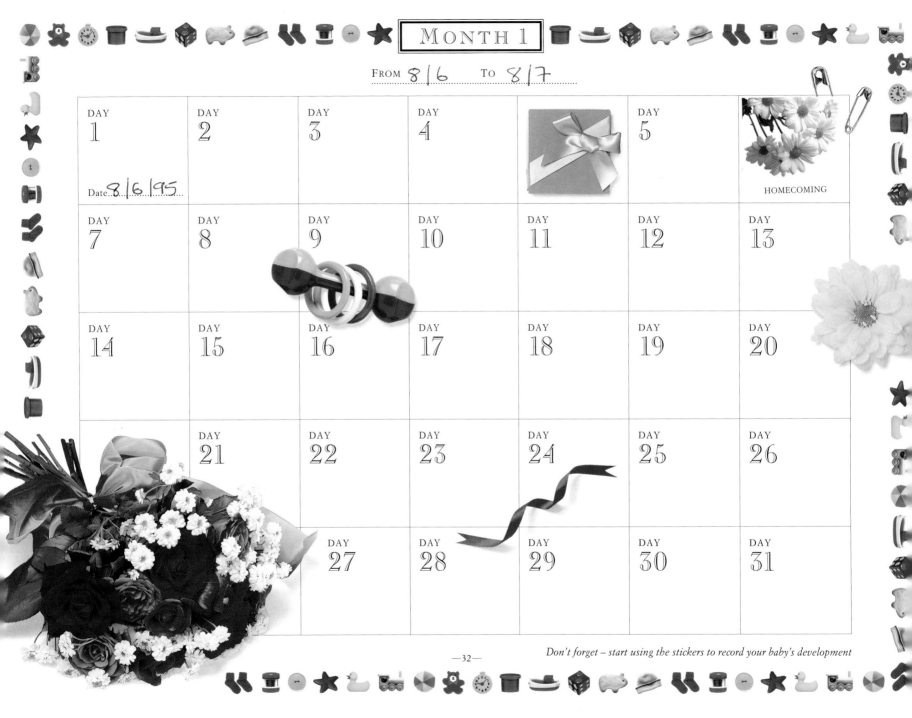

FROM .... TO ....

Weight ....

Length ....

Sleeping pattern ....
....

Bed time ....

Feeding pattern ....
....

Physical changes ....
....

Medical checks ....
....

New sounds ....
....

PHOTOGRAPH

Date of photograph ....

Response to mother ....

A typical day ....

Response to father ....

....

FROM .... TO ....

PHOTOGRAPH

Weight ....

Length ....

Sleeping pattern ....

....

Bed time ....

Feeding pattern ....

....

....

Physical changes ....

....

Medical checks ....

....

New sounds ....

Date of photograph ....

A typical day ....

Response to mother ....

....

Response to father ....

....

FROM .... TO ....

DAY 1	DAY 2	DAY 3	DAY 4	DAY 5	DAY 6	DAY 7
Date						
DAY 8	DAY 9	DAY 10	DAY 11	DAY 12	DAY 13	DAY 14
DAY 15	DAY 16	DAY 17	DAY 18	DAY 19	DAY 20	
DAY 21	DAY 22	DAY 23	DAY 24	DAY 25	DAY 26	
DAY 27	DAY 28	DAY 29	DAY 30	DAY 31		

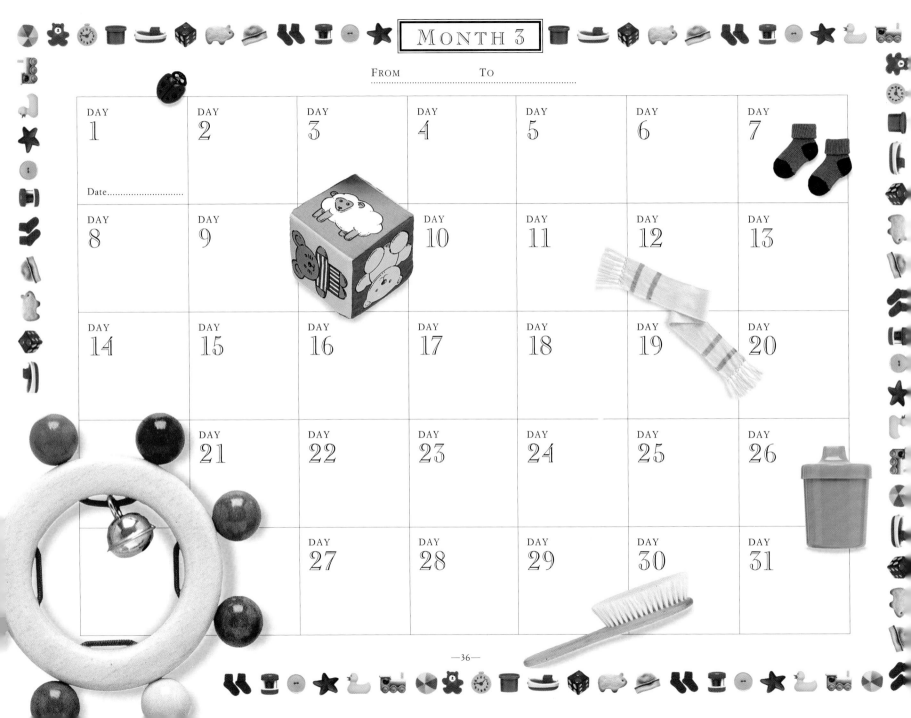

MONTH 3

FROM .... TO ....

DAY 1	DAY 2	DAY 3	DAY 4	DAY 5	DAY 6	DAY 7
Date............................						
DAY 8	DAY 9		DAY 10	DAY 11	DAY 12	DAY 13
DAY 14	DAY 15	DAY 16	DAY 17	DAY 18	DAY 19	DAY 20
	DAY 21	DAY 22	DAY 23	DAY 24	DAY 25	DAY 26
	DAY 27	DAY 28	DAY 29	DAY 30	DAY 31	

FROM .... TO ....

....

Weight .... Length ....

Sleeping pattern ....

....

Rises at ....

Bed time ....

Feeding pattern ....

Medical checks ....

....

Physical changes ....

....

New sounds ....

....

Response to mother ....

Response to father ....

A typical day ....

....

PHOTOGRAPH

Date of photograph

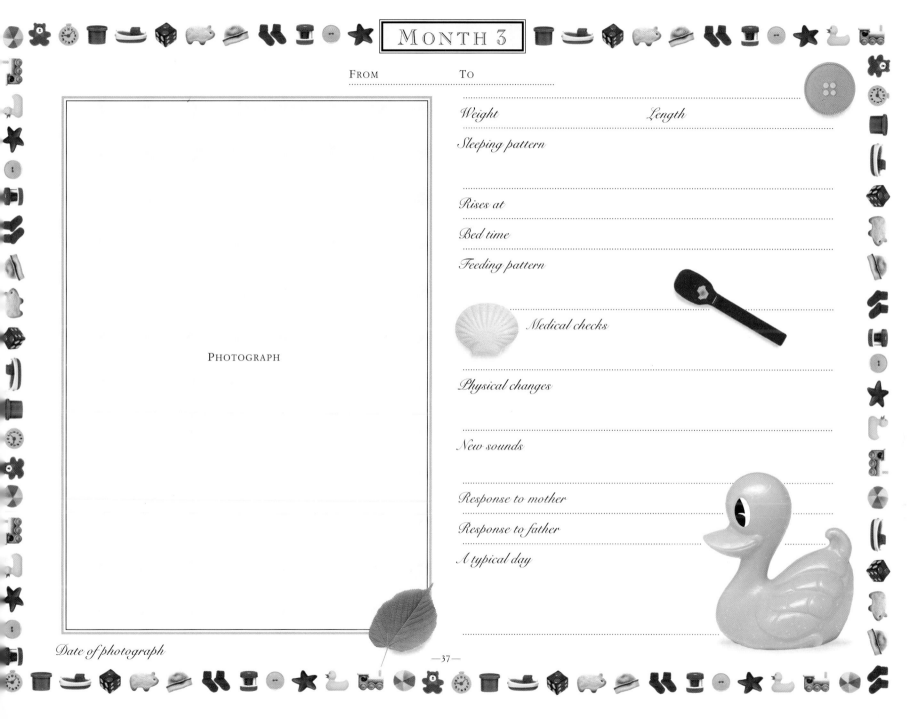

FROM .... TO ....

Weight .... Length ....

Sleeping pattern ....

Rises at ....

Bed time ....

Description of meal time ....

Physical changes ....

New movements ....

New sounds ....

Medical checks ....

Favourite activities ....

A typical day ....

PHOTOGRAPH

Date of photograph ....

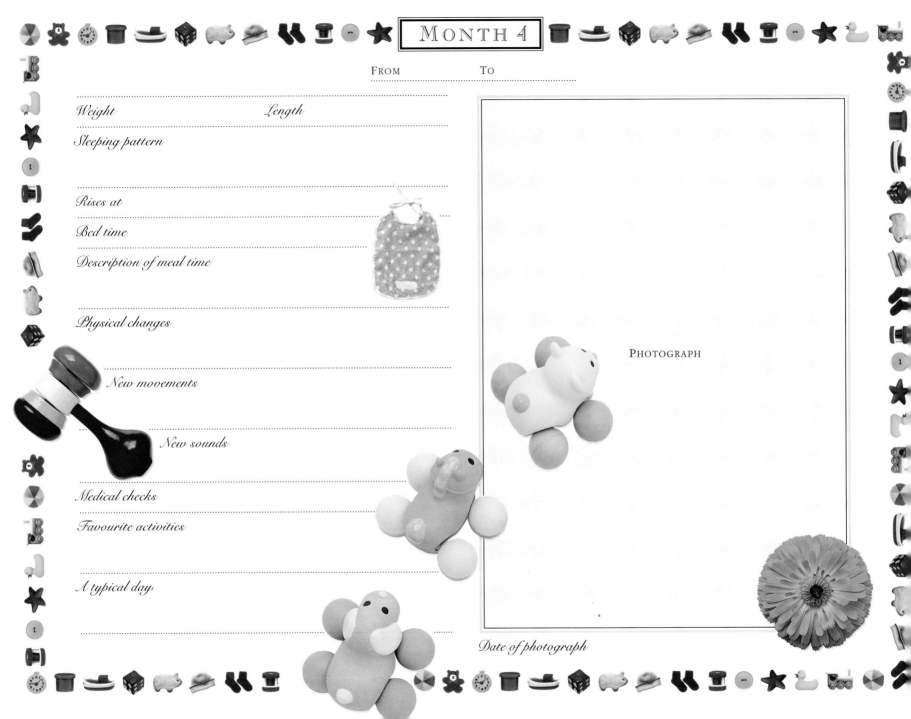

FROM .... TO ....

DAY 1	DAY 2	DAY 3	DAY 4	DAY 5	DAY 6	DAY 7
Date						
DAY 8	DAY 9	DAY 10	DAY 11	DAY 12	DAY 13	DAY 14
DAY 15	DAY 16	DAY 17	DAY 18			
DAY 19	DAY 20	DAY 21	DAY 22	DAY 23	DAY 24	
DAY 25	DAY 26	DAY 27	DAY 28	DAY 29	DAY 30	DAY 31

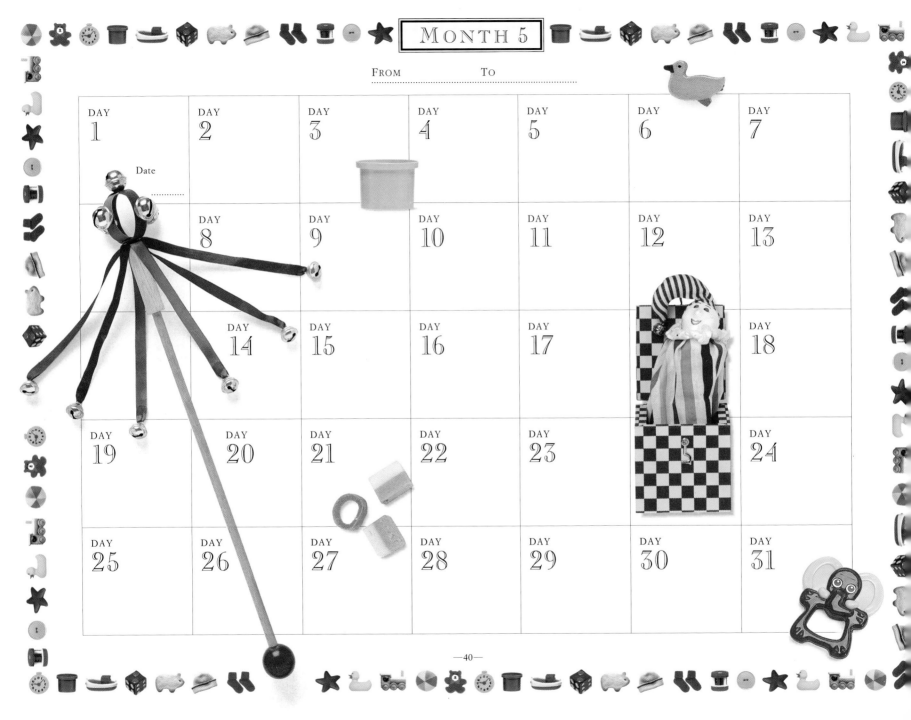

MONTH 5

FROM .... TO ....

DAY 1	DAY 2	DAY 3	DAY 4	DAY 5	DAY 6	DAY 7
Date	DAY 8	DAY 9	DAY 10	DAY 11	DAY 12	DAY 13
	DAY 14	DAY 15	DAY 16	DAY 17		DAY 18
DAY 19	DAY 20	DAY 21	DAY 22	DAY 23		DAY 24
DAY 25	DAY 26	DAY 27	DAY 28	DAY 29	DAY 30	DAY 31

—40—

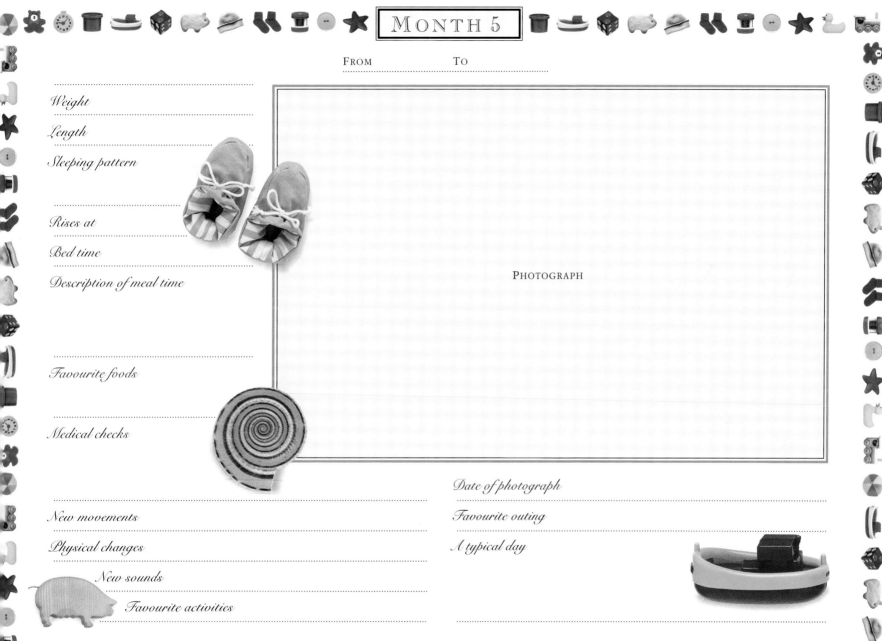

FROM .... TO ....

Weight ....

Length ....

Sleeping pattern ....

....

Rises at ....

Bed time ....

Description of meal time ....

....

Favourite foods ....

....

Medical checks ....

....

New movements ....

Physical changes ....

New sounds ....

Favourite activities ....

PHOTOGRAPH

Date of photograph ....

Favourite outing ....

A typical day ....

FROM .... TO ....

PHOTOGRAPH

Weight ....

Length ....

Sleeping pattern ....
....

Rises at ....

Bed time ....

Description of meal time ....
....

Favourite foods ....
....

Medical checks ....

Date of photograph ....

Favourite outing ....

A typical day ....

New movements ....

Physical changes ....

New sounds ....

Favourite activities ....

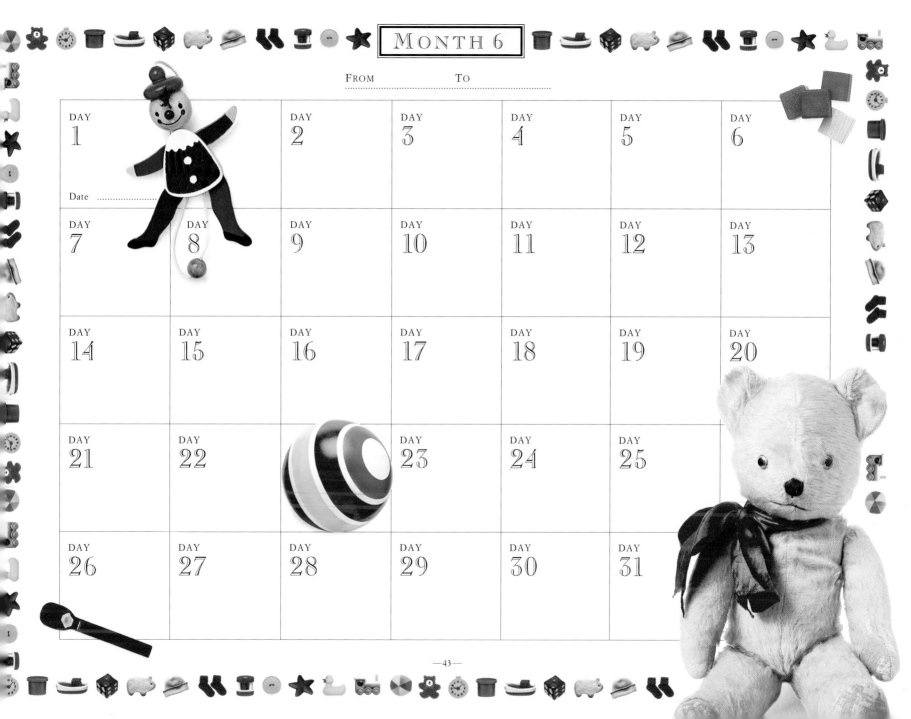

MONTH 6

FROM .... TO ....

DAY 1 Date	DAY 2	DAY 3	DAY 4	DAY 5	DAY 6
DAY 7	DAY 8	DAY 9	DAY 10	DAY 11	DAY 12	DAY 13
DAY 14	DAY 15	DAY 16	DAY 17	DAY 18	DAY 19	DAY 20
DAY 21	DAY 22	DAY 23	DAY 24	DAY 25
DAY 26	DAY 27	DAY 28	DAY 29	DAY 30	DAY 31

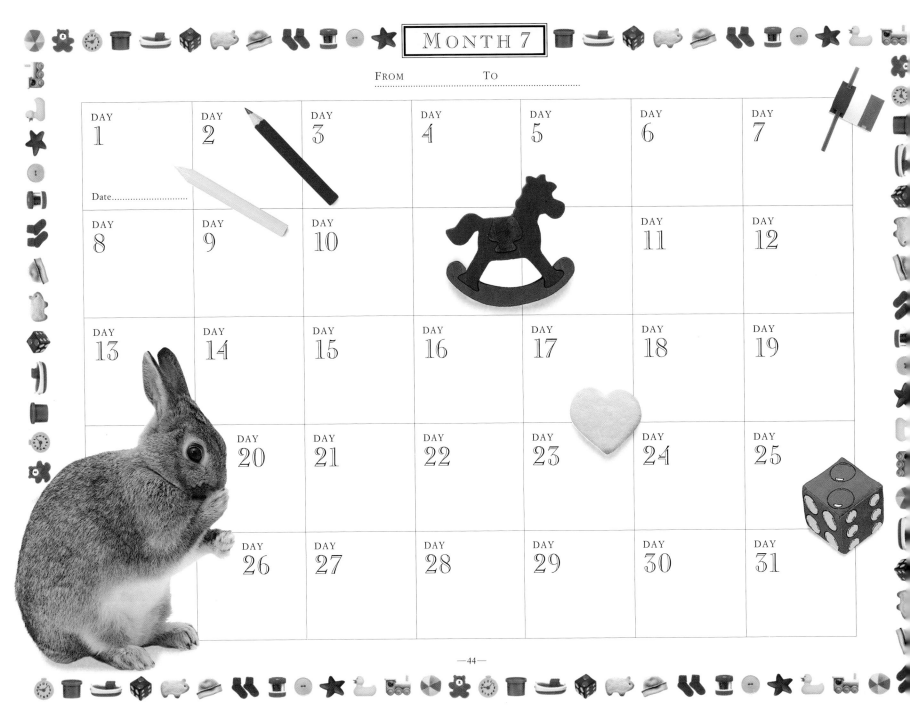

FROM _____ TO _____

DAY 1	DAY 2	DAY 3	DAY 4	DAY 5	DAY 6	DAY 7
Date...............	DAY 9	DAY 10			DAY 11	DAY 12
DAY 8						
DAY 13	DAY 14	DAY 15	DAY 16	DAY 17	DAY 18	DAY 19
			DAY 22	DAY 23	DAY 20	DAY 21
DAY 26	DAY 27	DAY 28	DAY 29	DAY 30	DAY 24	DAY 25
						DAY 31

FROM .... TO ....

Weight ....

Length ....

Sleeping pattern ....
....

Rises at ....

Bed time ....

Description of meal time ....
....

Favourite foods ....
....

Medical checks ....
....

New movements ....

Physical changes ....

New sounds ....

Favourite activities ....

PHOTOGRAPH

Date of photograph ....

Favourite outing ....

A typical day ....
....

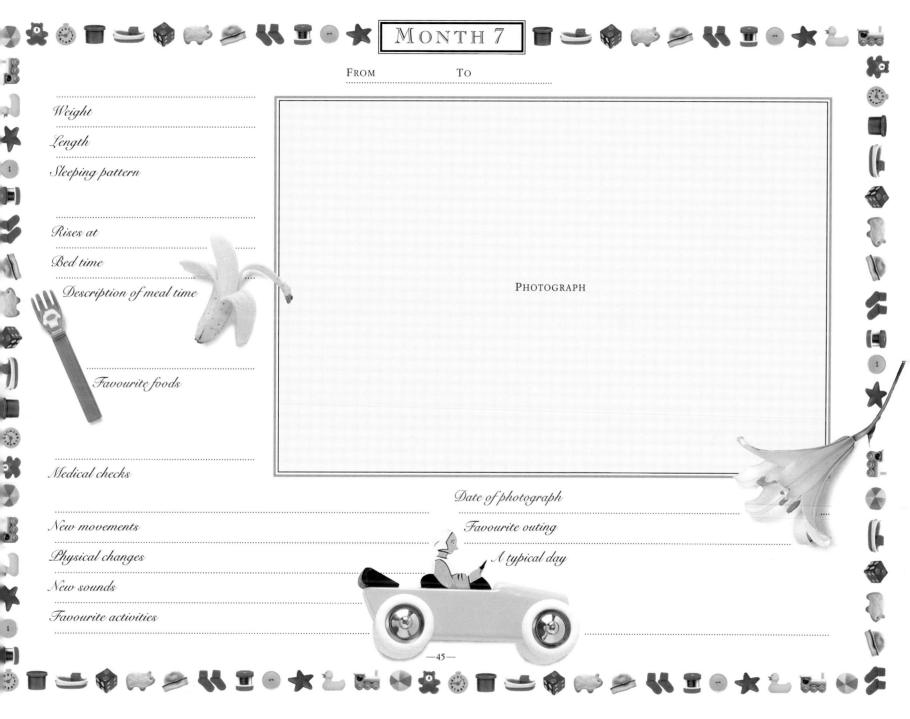

FROM .... TO ....

PHOTOGRAPH

Weight ....

Length ....

Sleeping pattern ....

Rises at ....

Bed time ....

Description of meal time ....

Favourite foods ....

Medical checks ....

Date of photograph ....

Favourite outing ....

A typical day ....

New movements ....

Physical changes ....

New sounds ....

Favourite activities ....

FROM   TO
....

DAY 1	DAY 2	DAY 3	DAY 4	DAY 5	DAY 6	DAY 7
Date						
DAY 8	DAY 9	DAY 10	DAY 11	DAY 12	DAY 13	DAY 14
DAY 15		DAY 16	DAY 17	DAY 18	DAY 19	DAY 20
DAY 21	DAY 22	DAY 23	DAY 24	DAY 25	DAY 26	
DAY 27	DAY 28	DAY 29	DAY 30	DAY 31		

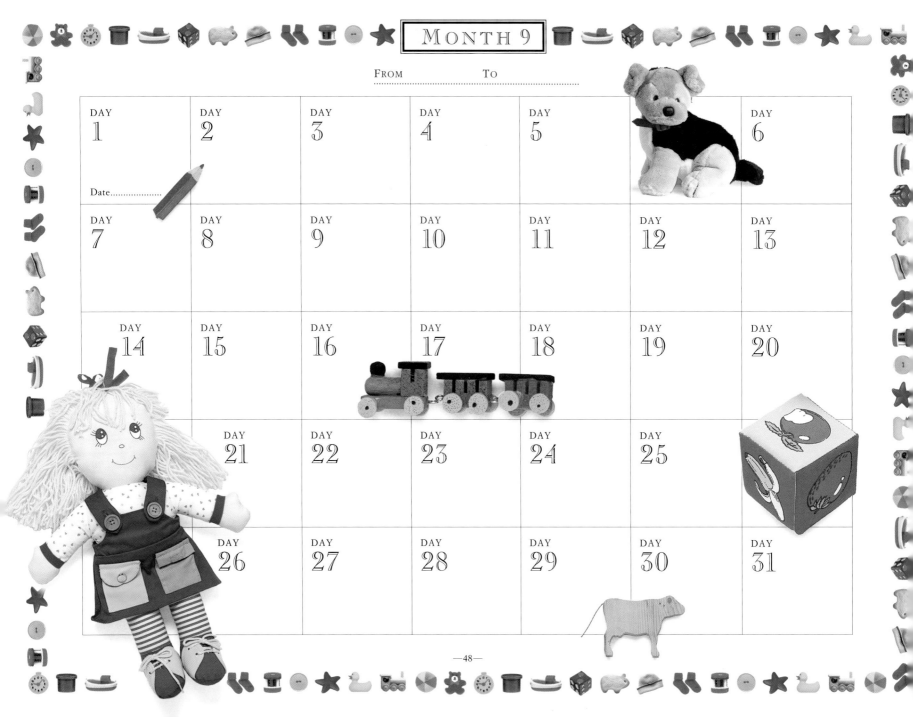

MONTH 9

FROM .... TO ....

DAY 1	DAY 2	DAY 3	DAY 4	DAY 5		DAY 6
Date...................	DAY 8	DAY 9	DAY 10	DAY 11	DAY 12	DAY 13
DAY 7						
DAY 14	DAY 15	DAY 16	DAY 17	DAY 18	DAY 19	DAY 20
	DAY 21	DAY 22	DAY 23	DAY 24	DAY 25	
	DAY 26	DAY 27	DAY 28	DAY 29	DAY 30	DAY 31

FROM .... TO ....

Weight .... Length ....

Sleeping pattern ....

Rises at ....

Bed time ....

Description of meal time ....

Physical changes ....

New movements ....

New sounds ....

Medical checks ....

Favourite activities ....

A typical day ....

PHOTOGRAPH

Date of photograph

MONTH 10

FROM .... TO ....

Weight .... Length ....

Sleeping pattern
....
....

Rises at ....

Bed time ....

Description of meal time
....
....

Physical changes
....
....

New movements
....
....

New sounds
....
....

Medical checks ....

Favourite activities
....
....

A typical day
....
....

PHOTOGRAPH

Date of photograph

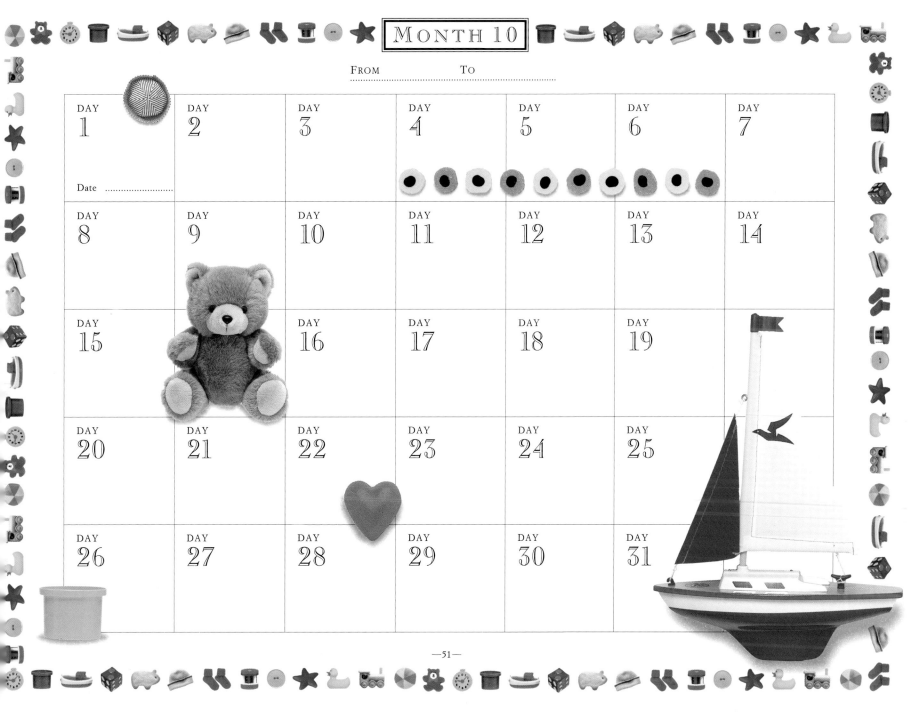

FROM .... TO ....

DAY 1	DAY 2	DAY 3	DAY 4	DAY 5	DAY 6	DAY 7
Date						
DAY 8	DAY 9	DAY 10	DAY 11	DAY 12	DAY 13	DAY 14
DAY 15		DAY 16	DAY 17	DAY 18	DAY 19	
DAY 20	DAY 21	DAY 22	DAY 23	DAY 24	DAY 25	
DAY 26	DAY 27	DAY 28	DAY 29	DAY 30	DAY 31	

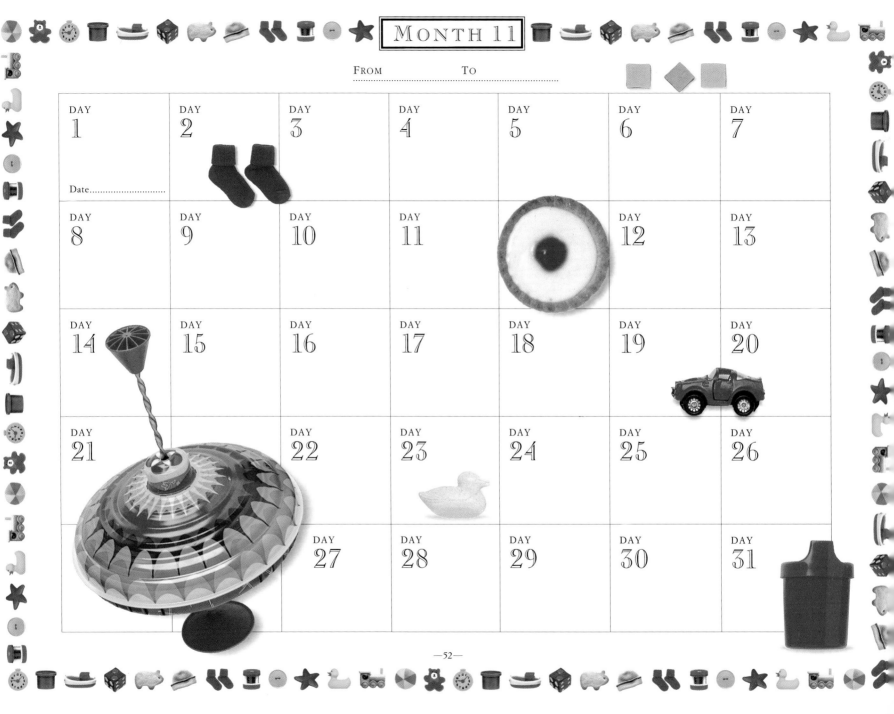

FROM .... TO ....

DAY 1

Date...........................

DAY 2

DAY 3

DAY 4

DAY 5

DAY 6

DAY 7

DAY 8

DAY 9

DAY 10

DAY 11

DAY 12

DAY 13

DAY 14

DAY 15

DAY 16

DAY 17

DAY 18

DAY 19

DAY 20

DAY 21

DAY 22

DAY 23

DAY 24

DAY 25

DAY 26

DAY 27

DAY 28

DAY 29

DAY 30

DAY 31

FROM .... TO ....

Weight ....

Length ....

Sleeping pattern ....

....

Rises at ....

Bed time ....

Description of meal time ....

Favourite foods ....

....

Medical checks ....

New movements ....

Physical changes ....

New sounds ....

Favourite activities ....

PHOTOGRAPH

Date of photograph ....

Favourite outing ....

A typical day ....

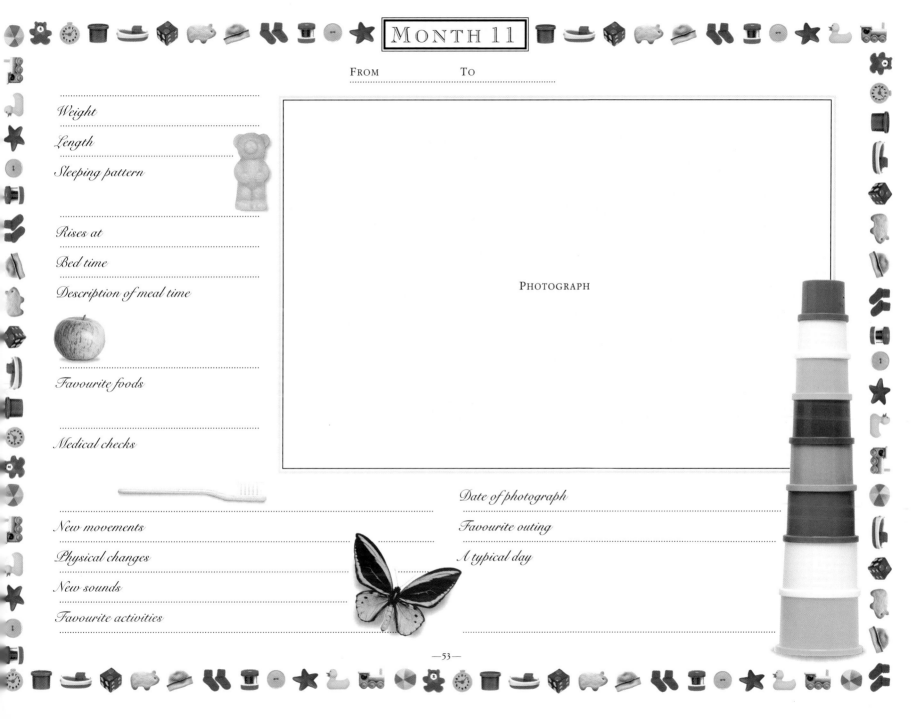

FROM .... TO ....

PHOTOGRAPH

Weight ....

Length ....

Sleeping pattern ....
....

Rises at ....

Bed time ....

Description of meal time ....
....

Favourite foods ....
....

Medical checks ....
....

Date of photograph ....

Favourite outing ....

A typical day ....

New movements ....

Physical changes ....

New sounds ....

Favourite activities ....

—54—

MONTH 12

FROM .... TO ....

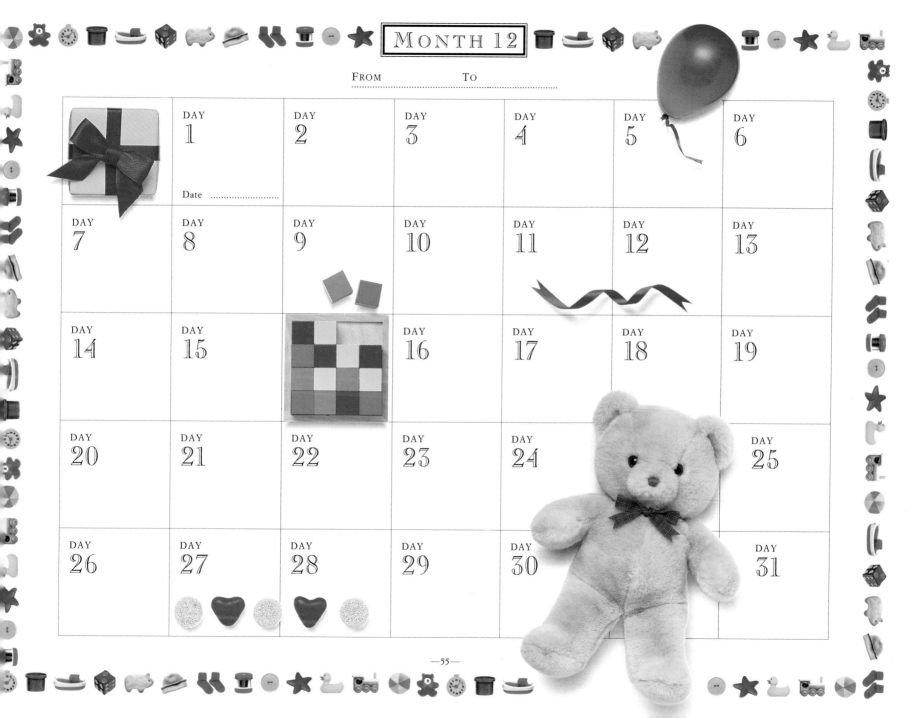	DAY 1 Date	DAY 2	DAY 3	DAY 4	DAY 5	DAY 6
DAY 7	DAY 8	DAY 9	DAY 10	DAY 11	DAY 12	DAY 13
DAY 14	DAY 15	DAY 16	DAY 17	DAY 18	DAY 19
DAY 20	DAY 21	DAY 22	DAY 23	DAY 24	DAY 25
DAY 26	DAY 27	DAY 28	DAY 29	DAY 30	DAY 31

A Dorling Kindersley book

Design Bernard Higton
Text Caroline Ash

First published in Great Britain in 1995 by
Dorling Kindersley Limited,
9 Henrietta Street, London WC2E 8PS

A CIP catalogue record for this book is available
from the British Library

ISBN 0 7513 0179 5

Colour reproduction by Colourscan, Singapore
Printed and bound in China by Imago

Photography Stephen Oliver, Guy Ryecart,
Colin Keates Natural History Museum,
D K Studio

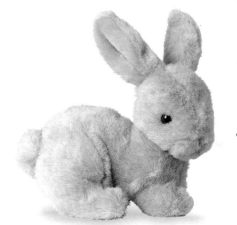

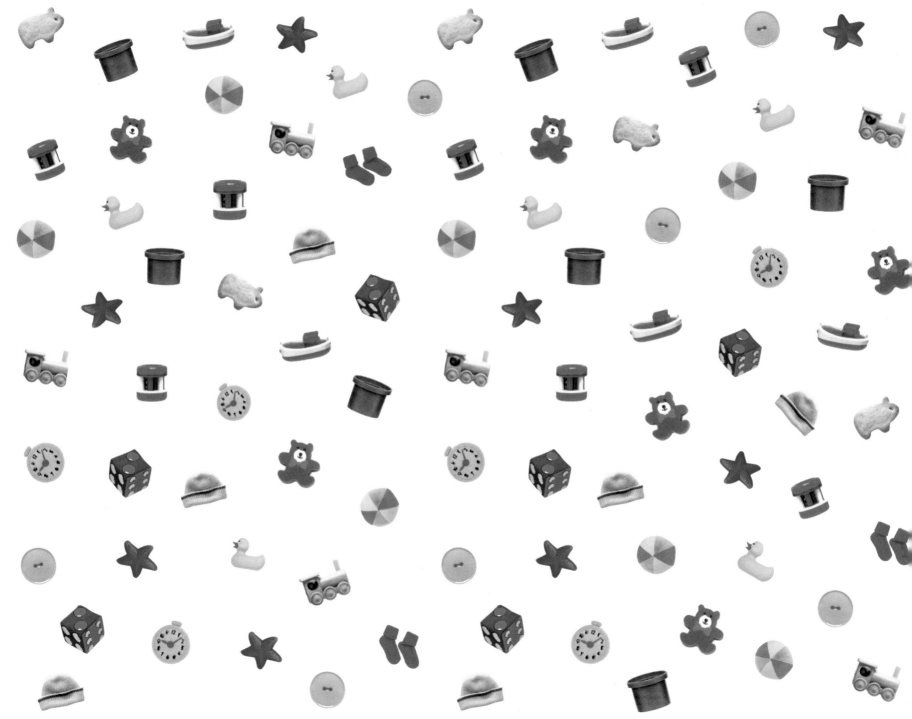

Baby RECORD BOOK STICKERS

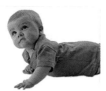

FIRST SMILE

HOLDS HEAD UP

HOLDS OBJECT

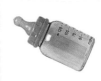

SITS UP

FIRST BOTTLE

FIRST KISS

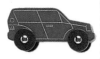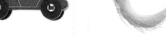

FIRST OUTING

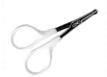

FIRST HAIRCUT

FIRST NAIL TRIM

FIRST SOLID FOOD

USES BEAKER

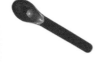

EATS WITH SPOON

EATS AT TABLE

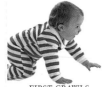

FIRST CRAWLS

FIRST TOOTH

FIRST BIG BATH

FIRST SLEEPS
THROUGH NIGHT

FIRST SLEEPS
IN COT

WAVES GOODBYE

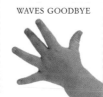

FIRST WORD

FIRST PARTY

FIRST RELIGIOUS
CEREMONY

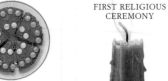

FIRST HOLIDAY

FIRST BABYSITTER

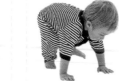

STANDS ALONE

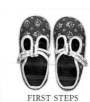

FIRST STEPS

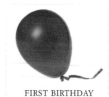

FIRST BIRTHDAY

FIRST VISIT TO
DOCTOR

VACCINATION

VACCINATION

VACCINATION

VACCINATION

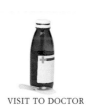

VISIT TO DOCTOR

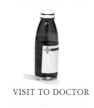

VISIT TO DOCTOR